BLOOD PRESSURE DIARY

**Make a lucid table of measured values,
both for yourself and presentation to your doctor.**

Contains <u>all</u> relevant data – systole, diastole, pulse, as well as **pulse pressure** and **arrhythmia detection**. With date, time, **place of measurement**, and notes.

Take your measurements only after a certain period of rest; this depends, of course, on the preceding activity. Stress situations and their reduction also influence blood pressure, among other factors.

All supplementary information in the book on blood pressure values and other are purely informative and do not constitute medical advice and are without claim to correctness. Only the qualified medical sector is the proper source of information and the right place to contact, also considering individual aspects of the patient as well as the latest findings and developments.

Personal Notes

Name: _____

_____

_____

_____

_____

_____

_____

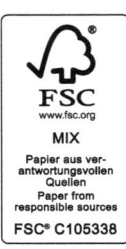

Bibliographic information published by the Deutsche Nationalbibliothek:
The Deutsche Nationalbibliothek lists this publication in the
Deutsche Nationalbibliografie; detailed bibliographic data
are available on the Internet at http://dnb.dnb.de

Printed and published by:
BoD - Books on Demand, Norderstedt

July 2022, 2nd edition

ISBN 9 783756 230723

This blood pressure diary contains not only the usual standard columns like date, time, systole, diastole, pulse, and notes, but includes three other important values for recording.

These are:

1. The **pulse pressure** (blood pressure amplitude). Already for some time, this has become an essential indicator, displayed separately on new devices. It is just a simple subtraction (upper minus lower blood pressure value) and can easily be calculated by yourself, especially when using older devices without this separate indication, but it should always be recorded.

2. Better devices also have an additional **arrhythmia detection** and can indicate cardiac arrhythmias. However, this is NOT a diagnosis of atrial fibrillation, replacing a professional medical examination, it merely indicates the POSSIBILITY of its presence. This can also be recorded in this booklet. In such a case, you should take a new measurement after a while, excluding possible measurement errors. Besides seeing the doctor, the device itself should be checked in case the suspicion is not confirmed.

3. It is also good to indicate the **measuring point** (upper arm or wrist), especially if you are using or trying out multiple devices on the arm or wrist. This can also be noted. If the measuring is always in the same place or unchanged over a longer period, it is sufficient to make only <u>one</u> entry, at the beginning of each double-page or on the day (hour) of changing the device – upper arm left/right UL, UR, or the wrist left/right WL, WR.

Remember, only the doctor can make reliable statements about particular parameters and individual target values, also taking into account individual circumstances (age etc.) and medications.

Do not rely merely on the many articles appearing on the Internet or in general-interest magazines. In addition, opinions and assessments, scientifically based or 'fudged', often change.

Especially with so many measuring devices of different qualities on the market (also taking into account a possibly necessary calibration), an occasional comparison when seeing your doctor is recommended. Also, pharmacists can take such measurements, following professional methods and specifications.

This booklet primarily serves the clear and complete recording of blood pressure measurements. Classifications and standards as well as supplementary statements and explanations have to come from the medical sector. Information contained herein is only of general nature without claim to correctness – especially concerning longer-term validness.

Moreover, the published values are not 'set in stone' for all eternity and are discussed again and again. Opinions also differ on whether target values should be achieved 'by hook or by crook' or whether a more moderate approach should be taken. The same applies to the general assessment of high blood pressure, where we have opinions saying that a treatment *strictly guidelines-oriented* might bear substantial risks, especially for older patients.

Hypotension = low blood pressure
Hypertension = high blood pressure

To write down guidelines or standards in such a nonmedical booklet makes no sense; therefore, just as an indication:

Blood pressure values (adults) published by the WHO – World Health Organization (2022). It should also be noted that there are differences according to age.

Categories	Systolic/ top value	Diastolic/ bottom value
Optimal	below 120	below 80
Normal	120 – 129	80 – 84
High normal	130 – 139	85 – 89
Grade-1-Hypertention (light)	140 – 159	90 – 99
Grade-2-Hypertention (advanced)	160 - 179	100 - 109
Grade-3-Hypertention (severe)	≥ 180	≥ 110

Low blood pressure (hypotension) is a variant eventually also needing treatment (but to be seen differently), ≤100/60 for men and ≤110/60 for women.

Pulse pressure – also a mere indication:

Normal	Elevated	High
under 55 mmHg	55 bis 65 mmHg	over 65 mmHg

Your own target values (best to use a pencil for possible later corrections):

Systole	Diastole	Pulse Pressure (lower than)

Date	Time	Systole (upper)	Diastole (lower)	Pulse	Pulse-Press.	A (1)	M (2)	Remarks

A **(1)** Indication of arrhythmia (heart rhythm disturbances). Leave free or write 'Yes' and make a new measurement after a break to exclude a false indication, otherwise consult a doctor without fail. Eventually, the measuring device has to be checked. M **(2)** =UL–upper arm left, UR–upper arm right, WL–wrist left, WR–wrist right.

Date	Time	Systole (upper)	Diastole (lower)	Pulse	Pulse-Press.	A (1)	M (2)	Remarks

Date	Time	Systole (upper)	Diastole (lower)	Pulse	Pulse-Press.	A (1)	M (2)	Remarks

A **(1)** Indication of arrhythmia (heart rhythm disturbances). Leave free or write 'Yes' and make a new measurement after a break to exclude a false indication, otherwise consult a doctor without fail. Eventually, the measuring device has to be checked. M **(2)** =UL–upper arm left, UR–upper arm right, WL–wrist left, WR–wrist right.

Date	Time	Systole (upper)	Diastole (lower)	Pulse	Pulse-Press.	A (1)	M (2)	Remarks

Date	Time	Systole (upper)	Diastole (lower)	Pulse	Pulse-Press.	A (1)	M (2)	Remarks

A **(1)** Indication of arrhythmia (heart rhythm disturbances). Leave free or write 'Yes' and make a new measurement after a break to exclude a false indication, otherwise consult a doctor without fail. Eventually, the measuring device has to be checked. M **(2)** =UL–upper arm left, UR–upper arm right, WL–wrist left, WR–wrist right.

Date	Time	Systole (upper)	Diastole (lower)	Pulse	Pulse-Press.	A (1)	M (2)	Remarks

Date	Time	Systole (upper)	Diastole (lower)	Pulse	Pulse-Press.	A (1)	M (2)	Remarks

A **(1)** Indication of arrhythmia (heart rhythm disturbances). Leave free or write 'Yes' and make a new measurement after a break to exclude a false indication, otherwise consult a doctor without fail. Eventually, the measuring device has to be checked. M **(2)** =UL–upper arm left, UR–upper arm right, WL–wrist left, WR–wrist right.

Date	Time	Systole (upper)	Diastole (lower)	Pulse	Pulse-Press.	A (1)	M (2)	Remarks

Date	Time	Systole (upper)	Diastole (lower)	Pulse	Pulse-Press.	A (1)	M (2)	Remarks

A **(1)** Indication of arrhythmia (heart rhythm disturbances). Leave free or write 'Yes' and make a new measurement after a break to exclude a false indication, otherwise consult a doctor without fail. Eventually, the measuring device has to be checked. M **(2)** =UL–upper arm left, UR–upper arm right, WL–wrist left, WR–wrist right.

Date	Time	Systole (upper)	Diastole (lower)	Pulse	Pulse-Press.	A (1)	M (2)	Remarks

Date	Time	Systole (upper)	Diastole (lower)	Pulse	Pulse-Press.	A (1)	M (2)	Remarks

A **(1)** Indication of arrhythmia (heart rhythm disturbances). Leave free or write 'Yes' and make a new measurement after a break to exclude a false indication, otherwise consult a doctor without fail. Eventually, the measuring device has to be checked. M **(2)** =UL–upper arm left, UR–upper arm right, WL–wrist left, WR–wrist right.

Date	Time	Systole (upper)	Diastole (lower)	Pulse	Pulse-Press.	A (1)	M (2)	Remarks

Date	Time	Systole (upper)	Diastole (lower)	Pulse	Pulse-Press.	A **(1)**	M **(2)**	Remarks

A **(1)** Indication of arrhythmia (heart rhythm disturbances). Leave free or write 'Yes' and make a new measurement after a break to exclude a false indication, otherwise consult a doctor without fail. Eventually, the measuring device has to be checked. M **(2)** =UL–upper arm left, UR–upper arm right, WL–wrist left, WR–wrist right.

Date	Time	Systole (upper)	Diastole (lower)	Pulse	Pulse-Press.	A (1)	M (2)	Remarks

Date	Time	Systole (upper)	Diastole (lower)	Pulse	Pulse-Press.	A (1)	M (2)	Remarks

A (1) Indication of arrhythmia (heart rhythm disturbances). Leave free or write 'Yes' and make a new measurement after a break to exclude a false indication, otherwise consult a doctor without fail. Eventually, the measuring device has to be checked. M (2) =UL–upper arm left, UR–upper arm right, WL–wrist left, WR–wrist right.

Date	Time	Systole (upper)	Diastole (lower)	Pulse	Pulse-Press.	A (1)	M (2)	Remarks

Date	Time	Systole (upper)	Diastole (lower)	Pulse	Pulse-Press.	A (1)	M (2)	Remarks

A **(1)** Indication of arrhythmia (heart rhythm disturbances). Leave free or write 'Yes' and make a new measurement after a break to exclude a false indication, otherwise consult a doctor without fail. Eventually, the measuring device has to be checked. M **(2)** =UL-upper arm left, UR-upper arm right, WL-wrist left, WR-wrist right.

Date	Time	Systole (upper)	Diastole (lower)	Pulse	Pulse-Press.	A (1)	M (2)	Remarks

Date	Time	Systole (upper)	Diastole (lower)	Pulse	Pulse-Press.	A (1)	M (2)	Remarks

A **(1)** Indication of arrhythmia (heart rhythm disturbances). Leave free or write 'Yes' and make a new measurement after a break to exclude a false indication, otherwise consult a doctor without fail. Eventually, the measuring device has to be checked. M **(2)** =UL–upper arm left, UR–upper arm right, WL–wrist left, WR–wrist right.

Date	Time	Systole (upper)	Diastole (lower)	Pulse	Pulse-Press.	A (1)	M (2)	Remarks

Date	Time	Systole (upper)	Diastole (lower)	Pulse	Pulse-Press.	A (1)	M (2)	Remarks

A **(1)** Indication of arrhythmia (heart rhythm disturbances). Leave free or write 'Yes' and make a new measurement after a break to exclude a false indication, otherwise consult a doctor without fail. Eventually, the measuring device has to be checked. M **(2)** =UL–upper arm left, UR–upper arm right, WL–wrist left, WR–wrist right.

Date	Time	Systole (upper)	Diastole (lower)	Pulse	Pulse-Press.	A (1)	M (2)	Remarks

Date	Time	Systole (upper)	Diastole (lower)	Pulse	Pulse-Press.	A (1)	M (2)	Remarks

A **(1)** Indication of arrhythmia (heart rhythm disturbances). Leave free or write 'Yes' and make a new measurement after a break to exclude a false indication, otherwise consult a doctor without fail. Eventually, the measuring device has to be checked. M **(2)** =UL–upper arm left, UR–upper arm right, WL–wrist left, WR–wrist right.

Date	Time	Systole (upper)	Diastole (lower)	Pulse	Pulse-Press.	A (1)	M (2)	Remarks

Date	Time	Systole (upper)	Diastole (lower)	Pulse	Pulse-Press.	A (1)	M (2)	Remarks

A **(1)** Indication of arrhythmia (heart rhythm disturbances). Leave free or write 'Yes' and make a new measurement after a break to exclude a false indication, otherwise consult a doctor without fail. Eventually, the measuring device has to be checked. M **(2)** =UL–upper arm left, UR–upper arm right, WL–wrist left, WR–wrist right.

Date	Time	Systole (upper)	Diastole (lower)	Pulse	Pulse-Press.	A (1)	M (2)	Remarks

Date	Time	Systole (upper)	Diastole (lower)	Pulse	Pulse-Press.	A (1)	M (2)	Remarks

A **(1)** Indication of arrhythmia (heart rhythm disturbances). Leave free or write 'Yes' and make a new measurement after a break to exclude a false indication, otherwise consult a doctor without fail. Eventually, the measuring device has to be checked. M **(2)** =UL–upper arm left, UR–upper arm right, WL–wrist left, WR–wrist right.

Date	Time	Systole (upper)	Diastole (lower)	Pulse	Pulse-Press.	A (1)	M (2)	Remarks

Date	Time	Systole (upper)	Diastole (lower)	Pulse	Pulse-Press.	A (1)	M (2)	Remarks

A **(1)** Indication of arrhythmia (heart rhythm disturbances). Leave free or write 'Yes' and make a new measurement after a break to exclude a false indication, otherwise consult a doctor without fail. Eventually, the measuring device has to be checked. M **(2)** =UL-upper arm left, UR-upper arm right, WL-wrist left, WR-wrist right.

Date	Time	Systole (upper)	Diastole (lower)	Pulse	Pulse-Press.	A (1)	M (2)	Remarks

Date	Time	Systole (upper)	Diastole (lower)	Pulse	Pulse-Press.	A (1)	M (2)	Remarks

A **(1)** Indication of arrhythmia (heart rhythm disturbances). Leave free or write 'Yes' and make a new measurement after a break to exclude a false indication, otherwise consult a doctor without fail. Eventually, the measuring device has to be checked. M **(2)** =UL–upper arm left, UR–upper arm right, WL–wrist left, WR–wrist right.

Date	Time	Systole (upper)	Diastole (lower)	Pulse	Pulse-Press.	A (1)	M (2)	Remarks

Date	Time	Systole (upper)	Diastole (lower)	Pulse	Pulse-Press.	A (1)	M (2)	Remarks

A **(1)** Indication of arrhythmia (heart rhythm disturbances). Leave free or write 'Yes' and make a new measurement after a break to exclude a false indication, otherwise consult a doctor without fail. Eventually, the measuring device has to be checked. M **(2)** =UL–upper arm left, UR–upper arm right, WL–wrist left, WR–wrist right.

Date	Time	Systole (upper)	Diastole (lower)	Pulse	Pulse-Press.	A (1)	M (2)	Remarks

Date	Time	Systole (upper)	Diastole (lower)	Pulse	Pulse-Press.	A (1)	M (2)	Remarks

A **(1)** Indication of arrhythmia (heart rhythm disturbances). Leave free or write 'Yes' and make a new measurement after a break to exclude a false indication, otherwise consult a doctor without fail. Eventually, the measuring device has to be checked. M **(2)** =UL–upper arm left, UR–upper arm right, WL–wrist left, WR–wrist right.

Date	Time	Systole (upper)	Diastole (lower)	Pulse	Pulse-Press.	A (1)	M (2)	Remarks

Date	Time	Systole (upper)	Diastole (lower)	Pulse	Pulse-Press.	A (1)	M (2)	Remarks

A **(1)** Indication of arrhythmia (heart rhythm disturbances). Leave free or write 'Yes' and make a new measurement after a break to exclude a false indication, otherwise consult a doctor without fail. Eventually, the measuring device has to be checked. M **(2)** =UL–upper arm left, UR–upper arm right, WL–wrist left, WR–wrist right.

Date	Time	Systole (upper)	Diastole (lower)	Pulse	Pulse-Press.	A (1)	M (2)	Remarks

Date	Time	Systole (upper)	Diastole (lower)	Pulse	Pulse-Press.	A (1)	M (2)	Remarks

A (1) Indication of arrhythmia (heart rhythm disturbances). Leave free or write 'Yes' and make a new measurement after a break to exclude a false indication, otherwise consult a doctor without fail. Eventually, the measuring device has to be checked. M (2) =UL–upper arm left, UR-upper arm right, WL-wrist left, WR-wrist right.

Date	Time	Systole (upper)	Diastole (lower)	Pulse	Pulse-Press.	A (1)	M (2)	Remarks

Date	Time	Systole (upper)	Diastole (lower)	Pulse	Pulse-Press.	A (1)	M (2)	Remarks

A (1) Indication of arrhythmia (heart rhythm disturbances). Leave free or write 'Yes' and make a new measurement after a break to exclude a false indication, otherwise consult a doctor without fail. Eventually, the measuring device has to be checked. M (2) =UL-upper arm left, UR-upper arm right, WL-wrist left, WR-wrist right.

Date	Time	Systole (upper)	Diastole (lower)	Pulse	Pulse-Press.	A (1)	M (2)	Remarks

Date	Time	Systole (upper)	Diastole (lower)	Pulse	Pulse-Press.	A (1)	M (2)	Remarks

A (1) Indication of arrhythmia (heart rhythm disturbances). Leave free or write 'Yes' and make a new measurement after a break to exclude a false indication, otherwise consult a doctor without fail. Eventually, the measuring device has to be checked. M (2) =UL–upper arm left, UR–upper arm right, WL–wrist left, WR–wrist right.

Date	Time	Systole (upper)	Diastole (lower)	Pulse	Pulse-Press.	A (1)	M (2)	Remarks

Date	Time	Systole (upper)	Diastole (lower)	Pulse	Pulse-Press.	A (1)	M (2)	Remarks

A **(1)** Indication of arrhythmia (heart rhythm disturbances). Leave free or write 'Yes' and make a new measurement after a break to exclude a false indication, otherwise consult a doctor without fail. Eventually, the measuring device has to be checked. M **(2)** =UL–upper arm left, UR–upper arm right, WL–wrist left, WR–wrist right.

Date	Time	Systole (upper)	Diastole (lower)	Pulse	Pulse-Press.	A (1)	M (2)	Remarks

Date	Time	Systole (upper)	Diastole (lower)	Pulse	Pulse-Press.	A (1)	M (2)	Remarks

A **(1)** Indication of arrhythmia (heart rhythm disturbances). Leave free or write 'Yes' and make a new measurement after a break to exclude a false indication, otherwise consult a doctor without fail. Eventually, the measuring device has to be checked. M **(2)** =UL–upper arm left, UR–upper arm right, WL–wrist left, WR–wrist right.

Date	Time	Systole (upper)	Diastole (lower)	Pulse	Pulse-Press.	A (1)	M (2)	Remarks

Date	Time	Systole (upper)	Diastole (lower)	Pulse	Pulse-Press.	A (1)	M (2)	Remarks

A **(1)** Indication of arrhythmia (heart rhythm disturbances). Leave free or write 'Yes' and make a new measurement after a break to exclude a false indication, otherwise consult a doctor without fail. Eventually, the measuring device has to be checked. M **(2)** =UL–upper arm left, UR–upper arm right, WL–wrist left, WR–wrist right.

Date	Time	Systole (upper)	Diastole (lower)	Pulse	Pulse-Press.	A (1)	M (2)	Remarks

Date	Time	Systole (upper)	Diastole (lower)	Pulse	Pulse-Press.	A (1)	M (2)	Remarks

A (1) Indication of arrhythmia (heart rhythm disturbances). Leave free or write 'Yes' and make a new measurement after a break to exclude a false indication, otherwise consult a doctor without fail. Eventually, the measuring device has to be checked. M (2) =UL–upper arm left, UR–upper arm right, WL–wrist left, WR–wrist right.

Date	Time	Systole (upper)	Diastole (lower)	Pulse	Pulse-Press.	A (1)	M (2)	Remarks

Date	Time	Systole (upper)	Diastole (lower)	Pulse	Pulse-Press.	A (1)	M (2)	Remarks

A **(1)** Indication of arrhythmia (heart rhythm disturbances). Leave free or write 'Yes' and make a new measurement after a break to exclude a false indication, otherwise consult a doctor without fail. Eventually, the measuring device has to be checked. M **(2)** =UL–upper arm left, UR–upper arm right, WL–wrist left, WR–wrist right.

Date	Time	Systole (upper)	Diastole (lower)	Pulse	Pulse-Press.	A (1)	M (2)	Remarks

Date	Time	Systole (upper)	Diastole (lower)	Pulse	Pulse-Press.	A (1)	M (2)	Remarks

A **(1)** Indication of arrhythmia (heart rhythm disturbances). Leave free or write 'Yes' and make a new measurement after a break to exclude a false indication, otherwise consult a doctor without fail. Eventually, the measuring device has to be checked. M **(2)** =UL–upper arm left, UR–upper arm right, WL–wrist left, WR–wrist right.

Date	Time	Systole (upper)	Diastole (lower)	Pulse	Pulse-Press.	A (1)	M (2)	Remarks

Date	Time	Systole (upper)	Diastole (lower)	Pulse	Pulse-Press.	A (1)	M (2)	Remarks

A **(1)** Indication of arrhythmia (heart rhythm disturbances). Leave free or write 'Yes' and make a new measurement after a break to exclude a false indication, otherwise consult a doctor without fail. Eventually, the measuring device has to be checked. M **(2)** =UL–upper arm left, UR–upper arm right, WL–wrist left, WR–wrist right.

Date	Time	Systole (upper)	Diastole (lower)	Pulse	Pulse-Press.	A (1)	M (2)	Remarks

Date	Time	Systole (upper)	Diastole (lower)	Pulse	Pulse-Press.	A (1)	M (2)	Remarks

A **(1)** Indication of arrhythmia (heart rhythm disturbances). Leave free or write 'Yes' and make a new measurement after a break to exclude a false indication, otherwise consult a doctor without fail. Eventually, the measuring device has to be checked. M **(2)** =UL–upper arm left, UR–upper arm right, WL–wrist left, WR–wrist right.

Date	Time	Systole (upper)	Diastole (lower)	Pulse	Pulse-Press.	A (1)	M (2)	Remarks

Date	Time	Systole (upper)	Diastole (lower)	Pulse	Pulse-Press.	A (1)	M (2)	Remarks

A **(1)** Indication of arrhythmia (heart rhythm disturbances). Leave free or write 'Yes' and make a new measurement after a break to exclude a false indication, otherwise consult a doctor without fail. Eventually, the measuring device has to be checked. M **(2)** =UL–upper arm left, UR–upper arm right, WL–wrist left, WR–wrist right.

Date	Time	Systole (upper)	Diastole (lower)	Pulse	Pulse-Press.	A (1)	M (2)	Remarks

Date	Time	Systole (upper)	Diastole (lower)	Pulse	Pulse-Press.	A (1)	M (2)	Remarks

A **(1)** Indication of arrhythmia (heart rhythm disturbances). Leave free or write 'Yes' and make a new measurement after a break to exclude a false indication, otherwise consult a doctor without fail. Eventually, the measuring device has to be checked. M **(2)** =UL–upper arm left, UR–upper arm right, WL–wrist left, WR–wrist right.

Date	Time	Systole (upper)	Diastole (lower)	Pulse	Pulse-Press.	A (1)	M (2)	Remarks

Date	Time	Systole (upper)	Diastole (lower)	Pulse	Pulse-Press.	A (1)	M (2)	Remarks

A **(1)** Indication of arrhythmia (heart rhythm disturbances). Leave free or write 'Yes' and make a new measurement after a break to exclude a false indication, otherwise consult a doctor without fail. Eventually, the measuring device has to be checked. M **(2)** =UL–upper arm left, UR–upper arm right, WL–wrist left, WR–wrist right.

Date	Time	Systole (upper)	Diastole (lower)	Pulse	Pulse-Press.	A (1)	M (2)	Remarks

Date	Time	Systole (upper)	Diastole (lower)	Pulse	Pulse-Press.	A (1)	M (2)	Remarks

A **(1)** Indication of arrhythmia (heart rhythm disturbances). Leave free or write 'Yes' and make a new measurement after a break to exclude a false indication, otherwise consult a doctor without fail. Eventually, the measuring device has to be checked. M **(2)** =UL–upper arm left, UR–upper arm right, WL–wrist left, WR–wrist right.

Date	Time	Systole (upper)	Diastole (lower)	Pulse	Pulse-Press.	A (1)	M (2)	Remarks

Date	Time	Systole (upper)	Diastole (lower)	Pulse	Pulse-Press.	A (1)	M (2)	Remarks

A (1) Indication of arrhythmia (heart rhythm disturbances). Leave free or write 'Yes' and make a new measurement after a break to exclude a false indication, otherwise consult a doctor without fail. Eventually, the measuring device has to be checked. M (2) =UL-upper arm left, UR-upper arm right, WL-wrist left, WR-wrist right.

Date	Time	Systole (upper)	Diastole (lower)	Pulse	Pulse-Press.	A (1)	M (2)	Remarks

Date	Time	Systole (upper)	Diastole (lower)	Pulse	Pulse-Press.	A (1)	M (2)	Remarks

A **(1)** Indication of arrhythmia (heart rhythm disturbances). Leave free or write 'Yes' and make a new measurement after a break to exclude a false indication, otherwise consult a doctor without fail. Eventually, the measuring device has to be checked. M **(2)** =UL–upper arm left, UR–upper arm right, WL–wrist left, WR–wrist right.

Date	Time	Systole (upper)	Diastole (lower)	Pulse	Pulse-Press.	A (1)	M (2)	Remarks

Date	Time	Systole (upper)	Diastole (lower)	Pulse	Pulse-Press.	A (1)	M (2)	Remarks

A **(1)** Indication of arrhythmia (heart rhythm disturbances). Leave free or write 'Yes' and make a new measurement after a break to exclude a false indication, otherwise consult a doctor without fail. Eventually, the measuring device has to be checked. M **(2)** =UL–upper arm left, UR–upper arm right, WL–wrist left, WR–wrist right.

Date	Time	Systole (upper)	Diastole (lower)	Pulse	Pulse-Press.	A (1)	M (2)	Remarks

Date	Time	Systole (upper)	Diastole (lower)	Pulse	Pulse-Press.	A (1)	M (2)	Remarks

A **(1)** Indication of arrhythmia (heart rhythm disturbances). Leave free or write 'Yes' and make a new measurement after a break to exclude a false indication, otherwise consult a doctor without fail. Eventually, the measuring device has to be checked. M **(2)** =UL–upper arm left, UR-upper arm right, WL–wrist left, WR–wrist right.

Date	Time	Systole (upper)	Diastole (lower)	Pulse	Pulse-Press.	A (1)	M (2)	Remarks

Date	Time	Systole (upper)	Diastole (lower)	Pulse	Pulse-Press.	A (1)	M (2)	Remarks

A **(1)** Indication of arrhythmia (heart rhythm disturbances). Leave free or write 'Yes' and make a new measurement after a break to exclude a false indication, otherwise consult a doctor without fail. Eventually, the measuring device has to be checked. M **(2)** =UL–upper arm left, UR–upper arm right, WL–wrist left, WR–wrist right.

Date	Time	Systole (upper)	Diastole (lower)	Pulse	Pulse-Press.	A (1)	M (2)	Remarks

Date	Time	Systole (upper)	Diastole (lower)	Pulse	Pulse-Press.	A (1)	M (2)	Remarks

A **(1)** Indication of arrhythmia (heart rhythm disturbances). Leave free or write 'Yes' and make a new measurement after a break to exclude a false indication, otherwise consult a doctor without fail. Eventually, the measuring device has to be checked. M **(2)** =UL–upper arm left, UR–upper arm right, WL–wrist left, WR–wrist right.

Date	Time	Systole (upper)	Diastole (lower)	Pulse	Pulse-Press.	A (1)	M (2)	Remarks

Date	Time	Systole (upper)	Diastole (lower)	Pulse	Pulse-Press.	A (1)	M (2)	Remarks

A **(1)** Indication of arrhythmia (heart rhythm disturbances). Leave free or write 'Yes' and make a new measurement after a break to exclude a false indication, otherwise consult a doctor without fail. Eventually, the measuring device has to be checked. M **(2)** =UL–upper arm left, UR–upper arm right, WL–wrist left, WR–wrist right.

Date	Time	Systole (upper)	Diastole (lower)	Pulse	Pulse-Press.	A (1)	M (2)	Remarks

Date	Time	Systole (upper)	Diastole (lower)	Pulse	Pulse-Press.	A (1)	M (2)	Remarks

A **(1)** Indication of arrhythmia (heart rhythm disturbances). Leave free or write 'Yes' and make a new measurement after a break to exclude a false indication, otherwise consult a doctor without fail. Eventually, the measuring device has to be checked. M **(2)** =UL–upper arm left, UR–upper arm right, WL–wrist left, WR–wrist right.

Date	Time	Systole (upper)	Diastole (lower)	Pulse	Pulse-Press.	A (1)	M (2)	Remarks

Date	Time	Systole (upper)	Diastole (lower)	Pulse	Pulse-Press.	A (1)	M (2)	Remarks

A (1) Indication of arrhythmia (heart rhythm disturbances). Leave free or write 'Yes' and make a new measurement after a break to exclude a false indication, otherwise consult a doctor without fail. Eventually, the measuring device has to be checked. M (2) = UL–upper arm left, UR–upper arm right, WL–wrist left, WR–wrist right.

Date	Time	Systole (upper)	Diastole (lower)	Pulse	Pulse-Press.	A (1)	M (2)	Remarks

Date	Time	Systole (upper)	Diastole (lower)	Pulse	Pulse-Press.	A (1)	M (2)	Remarks

A **(1)** Indication of arrhythmia (heart rhythm disturbances). Leave free or write 'Yes' and make a new measurement after a break to exclude a false indication, otherwise consult a doctor without fail. Eventually, the measuring device has to be checked. M **(2)** =UL-upper arm left, UR-upper arm right, WL-wrist left, WR-wrist right.

Date	Time	Systole (upper)	Diastole (lower)	Pulse	Pulse-Press.	A (1)	M (2)	Remarks